FINDING YOUR WAY OUT OF THE MENOPAUSE MAZE

*A 31 Day Devotional for
Kingdom-Minded Women*

TOPE PEARSON

Cover design by Ronna Fu
Flower image by Edyta of Patishop Art

To all my sisters-in-Christ;
daughters of the Most High God.
May you continue to be the princesses,
God has called you to be,
no matter what.

Index

ACKNOWLEDGMENTS

I would like to thank Anne Cunningham and Prue Bedwell for their care, advice and prayers concerning my health during this transition period. Thank you, Prue for endorsing this book. I am also grateful to Judith Spence, for her introduction of the likeness of the Church and the Proverbs 31 Woman.

I am especially thankful to my loving husband Tim Pearson, for his amazing support, especially during my trials.

Thank You Holy Spirit, for Your counsel and enabling me to write for the glory of the LORD.

INTRODUCTION

*I praise you because I am fearfully and wonderfully made; your works are wonderful,
I know that full well.*
PSALM 139:14

*"Your unique iris is proof that you are
God's handiwork."*
TOPE PEARSON

This pocket size daily devotional is written for women of God who are either going through or about to encounter your season of menopause. Menopause is a time in a woman's life when her body goes through changes in order to correct itself after regular menstruation cycles have ceased. Once you have gone twelve months without a period, you have reached menopause.

The average woman goes through menopause at age fifty one. The time period before menopause, is called perimenopause. This is not an easy time for most ladies but your Creator God knows, and is with you every day, hour, minute and second, as you try to figure out what is actually going on with your body, soul and spirit. As I mentioned in my previous booklet called, 'Heal to Health', God is love and we overcome by His grace. In your weakness, His power becomes perfect.

But he said to me, *"My grace is sufficient for you, for my power is made perfect in weakness."* Therefore, I will boast all the more gladly about my weaknesses, so that Christ's power may rest on me. 2 Corinthians 12:9

Going through hormonal changes can feel like being trapped in a maze, with no way out. It does not help if you are in environments where discussions about these issues are considered taboo, which can make you feel even more lost. Do not let the menopause process get you down or make you unfruitful, like the thorns in the Parable of the Sower (Matthew 13:22). Remember, it is only for a period in your life. Throughout this pocket book, I use the 'Proverbs 31 Woman' scenario, found in Proverbs 31:10 – 31, to give you hope on a daily basis. You can either see your glass as half empty or half full. So, for every thirty one menopause symptoms mentioned, I chose to see the opposite positive, and invite you to speak it out by faith. Jesus said, *"it is written…"* Use God's word – speak into the atmosphere and darkness must flee! Jesus' name is higher than menopause and all its symptoms, amen! In many scriptures when speaking about the 'wife' or 'bride,' it can symbolise the Church. I refer to this typification, in my book called 'The Wedding Dress'. So, remember you, as a born-again Christian, form part of the Body of Christ. Read Matthew 25 for example. Read also, Ephesians 5:23–33, especially verse 32. You have a specific call and purpose on earth, which the enemy would rather you get distracted and go into depression, to hinder the LORD's work through you. You are very needed at such a time as this (Esther 4:14). Who knows whether Queen Vasti was going through the menopause and missed a unique opportunity (see Esther 1)? In contrast, we know Naomi, who may have been at the age of menopause, managed to overcome her bitterness and depression, to see the fruit of her faith in God (Read the book of Ruth).

I hope you find the practical tips, scriptures, and prayers both healing and comforting. This is designed predominately for Kingdom-minded women, who feel they need a touch of God in specific areas of their well-being. It is your responsibility to check with your medical practitioner, before adhering to the practical tips which involve a change in diet or exercise. Press on towards your heavenly prize and do not allow this phase of your life to rob you of your peace and joy. Focus on serving Jesus Christ in these last days.

Consider it pure joy, my brothers and sisters, whenever you face trials of many kinds, because you know that the testing of your faith produces perseverance. James 1:2-3.

11

Day 1
Mood Swings, Sudden Tears &
Irritability .v. Character

"A wife of noble character who can find?"

Proverbs 31:10a

Hormonal changes can cause instant fluctuations in temperament and attitude, that you may not even recognise yourself in the moment. You can think you are losing the plot and wonder if your world is falling apart.

Your middle age, when experience, maturity, and wisdom is worn, could give way to pride, if not careful. It is important for women who walk with Godly confidence, to remember to decrease, so that Jesus may increase.

Consistent stress can be a key factor in exacerbating mood swings. Also, a lack of good diet, exercise, sleep, and iodine, play a significant part in the menopause symptoms.

As a woman of God, remember you are the Bride of Christ. Mood swings are not your portion – but Godly character; you do possess. You are capable, intelligent, and a virtuous woman; who is he who can find you? The enemy is scared of you and will try to attack your personality and reputation, but Jesus Christ has your back and never forgets the times when you have not been short with other people, or pushed them away in that moment. Know, Jesus has found you, because you belong to Him.

A PRACTICAL TIP:

Consider taking iodine supplements. Take a moment to reevaluate your life pattern. Reduce stress and be kind to yourself. When possible, go away for pamper treats and short holidays. Apologise to those you may have hurt and confide in those you trust. Fasting is key to overcome weaknesses. Sarah, Esther, and Naomi, despite their challenges, aired a noble character. It would be useful for you to study them in the Bible and see what helped them become the females God could use, despite their weaknesses.

A SHORT PRAYER:

My loving Father God, Thank You for the ability to discern the difference of when I am out of character and when there is a real issue which needs challenging. Please help me to possess the fruit of the Holy Spirit in every aspect of my life. I repent for hurting others and pray they will forgive me and bear with my weaknesses. In Jesus' name. Amen.

I decree and declare today: *"I am a woman of noble character.*

Day 2
Change in Body Odour & Weight Gain .v. Self-Worth

She is worth far more than rubies.

PROVERBS 31:10B

B ody odour changes are affected by the drop of estrogen levels that happens during the menopausal period. Excessive perspiration under the armpits and elsewhere can produce more bacteria, which causes unpleasant odour. Also, some experience bad breath due to a dry mouth condition which leave the mouth ripe for germs. Other symptoms such as dry tear duct, burning tongue, burning roof of mouth, and bad taste in mouth, gum problems, including increased bleeding can occur.

During menopause, low estrogen levels also promote fat storage in the belly area as visceral fat, which is linked to type 2 diabetes, heart disease, and other health problems.

Ladies obviously want to smell nice and can find unpleasant odours embarrassing; overweight uncomfortable and unattractive.

As a woman of God, remember you are the sweet

smelling aroma of Christ; you are treasured; you are far more precious than jewels and your value is far above rubies or pearls.

A PRACTICAL TIP:

Practice good hygiene, take natural supplements which include sage leaf, drink more water with sea salt (half teaspoon of unrefined sea salt for every ten glasses of water), engage in strength training to improve body composition, reduce carbs, eat a high fiber diet, visit your opticians for eye drops, and get good rest. If you are married, remember Abraham continued loving Sarah in her old age; likewise, Zachariah loved Elizabeth, the mother of John the Baptist. Do not be insecure about yourself. In God's arrangement, husbands are to love their wives and to cherish them (Ephesians 5:25). As his wife goes through the transition of menopause, a godly husband will make it his business to encourage her, because to him, she is worth it.

A SHORT PRAYER:

My loving Abba Father, thank You for making me who I am. Please show me how to look after my body well, which is the temple of the Hoy Spirit. But most of all, help me be secure in Your love. In Jesus' name. Amen.

I decree and declare today: "I am a woman of high value."

Day 3
Loss of Libido & Dry Vagina .v. Love & Affection

*Her husband has full confidence in her
and lacks nothing of value.*

Proverbs 31:11

Men-O-pause! You mean, take a pause from men?
Yes, let us face it ladies; it really does feel like
this at times. This can be a complex area of the marriage.
Sexual intercourse is only meant for married couples
(one man and one woman), as a gift from God. Many
women lose the urge to make love to their husbands
or to come to climax. Also, sexual intercourse can feel
uncomfortable and even painful due to dryness. This can
feel so discouraging that, eventually, you might decide
there is no point in trying, and give up entirely. Please do
not lose hope.

As a woman of God, whether you are single,
married, divorced, or widowed, remember Jesus' words:
*"The people of this age marry and are given in marriage. But
those who are considered worthy of taking part in the age to come
and in the resurrection from the dead will neither marry nor be*

given in marriage, and they can no longer die; for they are like the angels. They are God's children, since they are children of the resurrection…", Luke 20:34-37.

If, however, you are married, remember you are still loved by your husband, who should be trying to be sensitive to these changes, and show you affection. The heart of your husband (Jesus) trusts in you (the Church) confidently and relies on and believes in you securely, so that he has no lack of gain. His eyes and heart is stayed on the one he married; the one he chose to be his soul-mate; to love and to hold; for better or for worse; until death, or the return of Jesus Christ, our eternal Bridegroom.

A PRACTICAL TIP:

Scripture states: *"Do not deprive each other except perhaps by mutual consent and for a time, so that you may devote yourselves to prayer. Then come together again so that Satan will not tempt you because of your lack of self-control",* 1 Corinthians 7:5. Therefore, write down thirty-one good qualities and things you like about your husband. Meditate on each one per day throughout this 31-day devotional. Think of the moments, especially, when that particular good characteristic occurred and when he made you laugh, feel secure and cherished. Remember your husband is not perfect also, and needs forgiving when he gets it wrong.

Another solution is to try spending more time on erogenous play and non-physical intimacy. This does not just increase your arousal; it can also help you feel more connected to your husband.

Try applying a small dose of natural menopause cream (containing wild yam) on certain parts of your body as instructed. This can help restore vaginal fluid and increase your libido. You also cannot go wrong with a dash of good old fashioned petroleum jelly down below.

If you are really struggling in this area, to the point of serious marriage difficulties, endeavour to seek professional help, including Christian marriage counselling.

A SHORT PRAYER:

Our Father God, Thank You for my husband. Please help my husband to love me more; pray for me more, and be sensitive to my changes. Also help me to feel secure and not believe the lies of the enemy. In Jesus' name. Amen.

I decree and declare today: *"I am a woman who has the full confidence of my husband."*

DAY 4
FEELINGS OF DREAD & DOOM .V. FAITH

*She brings him good, not harm,
all the days of her life.*

PROVERBS 31:12

As women go through the menopausal journey, they experience a decline in estrogen levels, which lead to higher cortisol levels, that can disrupt the delicate balance in the brain. Reduced estrogen levels have therefore, been associated with increased feelings of anxiousness. Anxiety is how the body prepares to respond to a stressful situation or threat. It readies you for fight or flight. Have you been wondering why you may have recently developed into a bad passenger-driver; constantly feeling the car is going to crash? Or do you dwell on other unlikely events and disasters?

The reality is the potential damage you could cause yourself and others due to over-thinking. The wrong type of fear is found in punishment, 1 John 4:18. This can be disheartening, especially if you are in a position of leadership. Do not let the enemy rob your peace, as Jesus' plans are not to harm you, but prosper you, Jeremiah 29:11-13.

As a woman of God, remember doom is not around the corner, so there is no need to dread. Perfect love casts out fear, 1 John 4:18. God has got your back, and has not given you a spirit of fear but power, love, and a sound mind, 2 Timothy 1:7. The right type of fear is found in wisdom and that is to fear God alone! Deborah was a prophetess and a leader who strengthened Israel fearlessly, because she knew the God of Abraham, Isaac, and Jacob was her defender, Judges 4. As a woman of faith, therefore, you will comfort, encourage, and do only good to the Church, as long as there is life within you.

A PRACTICAL TIP:

Meditate on Philippians 4:4-8: *"Do not be anxious about anything, but in every situation, by prayer and petition, with thanksgiving, present your requests to God. And the peace of God, which transcends all understanding, will guard your hearts and your minds in Christ Jesus… [sisters], whatever is true, whatever is noble, whatever is right, whatever is pure, whatever is lovely, whatever is admirable—if anything is excellent or praiseworthy—think about such things."*

Physical activity helps divert your attention and triggers chemical changes in the brain that keep anxiety at bay.

Christian Cognitive-behavioral therapy (CBT): This form of talk therapy, if led by a qualified Christian

Counsellor, who incorporates pastoral care, could help you focus on changing thought and behavior patterns, helping you see anxiety-inducing situations more clearly and respond to them more healthily.

Join a mature Christian women's group, where you can be open, real and feel it is a safe space to share and pray for each other.

A SHORT PRAYER:

My Heavenly Father, thank You for Your word. Please increase my faith? Thank You for Your undying love and giving me eternal life, so that I may be salt and light for Christ; doing good wherever I go. In Jesus' name. Amen.

I decree and declare today: *"I am a woman of faith."*

DAY 5
BRITTLE & WEAK FINGERNAILS
.V. GRACE

She selects wool and flax
and works with eager hands

PROVERBS 31:13

Menopause transition can reduce your level of keratin, which is a protective protein in your body. Have you been questioning why your nails are softer and break easier than before?

Women use their hands for lots of chores, as we multitask our way through life. The issue is, we likewise want to be well-groomed to look presentable in our profession and social environment. It can be disheartening when you see your natural nails are not what they used to be, and the first thing you think of is to hide them under nail polish. Or you feel apprehensive to take on the usual tasks which tend to cause your nails to break.

As a woman of God, remember weaker nails will not distract you from your mission, as God's grace is sufficient for you, and in your weakness, His strength becomes perfect, 2 Corinthians 12:9. As a woman of grace, therefore, you seek out wool and flax (whatever the church has to hand) and works with willing hands to develop it.

A PRACTICAL TIP:

Keep hydrated, moisture your hands regularly, avoid using gel polish and false nails. Eat plenty iron-rich foods, including dark-green leafy vegetables.

A SHORT PRAYER:

Dear God, thank You for my beautiful hands. Please restore my keratin levels and help me not to allow my weaker nails to become a distraction from using my hands to eagerly work for You. In Jesus' name. Amen.

I decree and declare today: *"I am a woman of grace."*

Day 6
Indigestion, Gas Pain & Nausea .v. Spiritual Growth

She is like the merchant ships,
bringing her food from afar.

Proverbs 31:14

Bloating during perimenopause and menopause is common and may be the result of fluctuating hormones during this period of your life. You may wonder if you have over-eaten after each meal, but this may not always be the case.

Women who have gone through periods and pregnancy would be familiar with the pain of heart-burn and discomfort of nausea. You may even feel you are 'with-child' or the food you ate did not agree with you. Embarrassment comes with gas or uncontrollable wind and can make you want to self-isolate.

As a woman of God, remember you are expanding spiritually, and any pain you feel is the pruning of God, the Gardener in John 15:1-8. You are like the merchant ships loaded with foodstuff, that is, spiritual food; you bring your household's spiritual food from a far country.

You bring in resources like speakers and teaching material, from outside of your denomination or area, so your church can grow, Ephesians 4:11-16.

A PRACTICAL TIP:

Cut down on foods that are known to cause gas, like cabbage, beans or lentils and high processed sugary foods.

A SHORT PRAYER:

Dear God, thank You for my good health. Please heal my gut and help me to focus on strengthening the Body of Christ, and allow your pruning, so I can bear fruit that will last. In Jesus' name. Amen.

I decree and declare today: *"I am a woman who grows spiritually."*

Day 7

Trouble Sleeping through the Night .v. Intercession

She gets up while it is still night;
she provides food for her family
and portions for her female servants.

Proverbs 31:15

Insomnia is a sleeping disorder that prevents people from getting adequate sleep, and is a symptom related to menopause. You may feel like climbing the walls during night hours, even though you avoided caffeine and sugary foods all day.

Not getting enough sleep can make you feel more irritable, tired, tearful, and stressed. If you do not work with empathetic managers or colleagues, this could further exacerbate the other menopause symptoms and make you feel like giving up.

I urge you to keep on keeping on. As a woman of God, remember good sleep is your portion. However, when you rise while it is yet night and spiritually dark, you get your spiritual food first, for yourself, as woman cannot not live by bread alone, but by every word that proceeds from the mouth of God, Matthew 4:4. This then propels you to pray and intercede for your household and nation, and assign your bridesmaids, staff team, congregation, and volunteers, their tasks in joining with you to build the Body of Christ in making disciple-makers of all nations, Matthew 28:18-20.

A PRACTICAL TIP:

Before you sleep, drink herbal night tea, containing essential properties which aid with sleep. Lavinder oil rubbed onto your inner wrist can help, but first check for allergies. Keep your Bible, journal, and pen by your bedside. When you wake up, read, and meditate on God's word, especially Psalm 62:1-2; then be still and know He is God, Psalm 46:10. Practice relaxation techniques through soaking (i.e. laying down with your eyes closed, and heart focused on Jesus Christ, as you listen to gentle Christian praise and worship instrumental music).

A SHORT PRAYER:

Dear God, thank You for sleep. Please help me to get sufficient sleep, so I can fulfil the Great Commission. For I know, You will keep in perfect peace, those whose minds are steadfast, because they trust in you, Isaiah 26:3. In Jesus' name. Amen.

I decree and declare today: *"I am a woman of Intercessory prayer."*

DAY 8
DISTURBING MEMORY LAPSES
.V. INSIGHT

She considers a field and buys it;

PROVERBS 31:16A

Estrogen and progesterone loss on the brain can cause a type of memory loss linked to the menopause, sometimes described as brain fog. You might struggle to focus properly at work or feel unable to concentrate on your projects. You could also find it hard to remember peoples' names, or simply lose your keys more often.

Regular forgetfulness could give the impression to others that you are disregarding them or your work, or unconcerned about the situation or environment you find yourself in. For some women, it can lead to embarrassment and a loss of confidence.

As a woman of God, remember Jesus! His name is above all names! As long as you do not forget Jesus, you will use insight and consider and a new field; a physical or spiritual area for sowing and reaping before you buy or accept it. Expanding prudently and not courting neglect of your present duties by assuming other duties, Isaiah 54:2.

A PRACTICAL TIP:

Read more inspirational books, newspapers and magazines. Learn something new, play puzzle games or quizzes, and spend time socializing with family and friends.

A SHORT PRAYER:

Dear God, thank You for insight. Please help me to remember all I need to for work and life's responsibilities You have given me to steward, especially in the ministry of reconciliation. For I know, I have the mind of Christ, 1 Corinthians 2:16. In Jesus' name. Amen.

I decree and declare today: *"I am a woman of insight."*

DAY 9
DIFFICULTY CONCENTRATING & DISORIENTATION .V. FRUITFUL

..out of her earnings she plants a vineyard.

PROVERBS 31:16B

Mental confusion is similar to brain fog. At times, you may not know your location and identity, or the time and date. You may not be able to think with your normal level of clarity; even delirium, or having disrupted attention.

Other people may not understand what is happening to you and may doubt your ability to make sound decisions. This again can deplete your morale.

As a woman of God, remember you have order and are fruitful for Christ; the LORD has faith in you. You, by increasing, and with your savings (of time, finances, and strength), you plant fruitful vines in your vineyard, which includes individual souls, groups, congregations and nations, Psalm 2.

A PRACTICAL TIP:

Exercise your mind daily. Talk to trusted people if confusion gets severe. Go on the streets, or in your neighbourhood to witness for Jesus Christ. Join a mature Christian women's group, where you can support one another.

A SHORT PRAYER:

Dear God, thank You for making me fruitful. Please help me to remember all I need to for the work and purpose you have given me to steward. For I know, I have the mind of Christ, 1 Corinthians 2:16. In Jesus' name. Amen.

I decree and declare today: *"I am a woman of fruitfulness."*

DAY 10
CRASHING FATIGUE .V. INVIGORATE

She sets about her work vigorously

PROVERBS 31:17A

Menopause fatigue is often referred to as 'crushing'. It is a feeling of overwhelming, sudden 'crashing' tiredness, as though you are about to come down with a virus. Ever wondered why you often feel drained, even when you have had the recommended eight-hour sleep?

Constant tiredness can adversely affect your quality of life. As multi-taskers, women want to be productive in all we do. So, not being able to feel energised and refreshed to do your work and life, can be a little demoralising.

As a woman of God, remember, as an act of worship, you gird yourself with strength; spiritual, mental, and physical fitness, for your God-given task. You fan into flames the gifts within you, 2 Timothy 1:6. You work as though working for the LORD, as it is Christ you are serving, Colossians 3:24.

A PRACTICAL TIP:

Avoid eating heavy meals too close to bedtime and develop a good sleep routine. You may consider getting checked by a doctor or nurse to ensure you are not anemic.

A SHORT PRAYER:

Dear God, thank You for giving me the energy I need to fulfil Your purpose for my life, here on earth. I am looking forward to the glorious body You will give me, so I can serve You eternally during Your Millennium Reign! In Jesus' name. Amen.

I decree and declare today: *"I am a woman of vigor."*

Day 11
Aching, Sore Joints, Muscles & Tendons .v. Strength

her arms are strong for her tasks.

Proverbs 31:17b

Menopause may cause joint pain because as your levels of estrogen, which helps to reduce inflammation, declines, this causes discomfort and menopause-related arthritis may start to manifest. Muscle tension or spasm is another menopause symptom and can be extremely painful.

When your knees are feeble and ankles give way whilst walking or running, this can cause falls, hence further injuries. It could also slow down or limit the type of exercise you do, plus your work and life, through fear of hurting yourself.

As a woman of God, remember Christ make your arms strong and firm. You can do all things through Christ who strengthens you, Philippians 4:13.

A PRACTICAL TIP:

Watch your posture. Hold onto the bannisters when walking up and down stairs. Ice or heat packs can help reduce joint pain and inflammation. Wear knee or ankle sleeves if required. You could also wear lower back support. Avoid high impact exercise and try walking or swimming instead. Eat more fish with omega 3 fatty oils. Take Glucosamine supplements after consulting with your GP, as this might increase the cartilage and fluid around your joints and help prevent their breakdown.

A SHORT PRAYER:

Dear God, thank You for giving me the strength I need to fulfil my purpose. Please protect my body from injuries, for Your glory. In Jesus' name. Amen.

I decree and declare today: *"I am a woman of strength."*

DAY 12
ANXIETY & FEELING ILL AT EASE .V. PROSPERITY

She sees that her trading is profitable,

PROVERBS 31:18A

One of the menopause symptoms is an occasional or constant nervous feeling. Worry can become common place in your life, and even lead to panic attacks.

As lots of other changes are happening at once, you may feel you are going through a mid-life crisis. Grown up children leaving home; last minute pressure to have your first child or one more child; younger and vibrant people coming into the workplace and possible threat to your career; over-thinking your relationships and over concern about being left alone. This type of unease could hinder your successes in life, cause you to self-sabotage close relationships, and shake your emotional and financial security.

As a woman of God, remember you do not worry about today or tomorrow. You observe the birds of the air; they do not sow or reap or store away in barns, and yet your heavenly Father feeds them. You know you are much more valuable than they, Matthew 6:25-27. You taste and perceive that your gain from work, with and for God, is good and you will prosper in mind and spirit, 3 John 2.

A PRACTICAL TIP:

Listen to calming Christian instrumental music and change your daily life-style to reduce stress. Practice five minutes daily of taking deep slow breaths from the abdomen.

A SHORT PRAYER:

Dear God, thank You for giving me prosperity. I pray that I may enjoy good health and that all may go well with me, even as my soul is getting along well. In Jesus' name. Amen.

I decree and declare today: *"I am a woman of prosperity."*

Day 13
Hot Flushes, Clammy & Night Sweats .v. Salt & Light

and her lamp does not go out at night.

PROVERBS 31:18B

Two of the most well-known and experienced signs of the menopause are known as vasomotor symptoms. You may feel an intense heat spread over your body and become flushed, often followed by sweating.

Have you ever woken up in a swimming pool during the middle of the night? Well, it can feel like that at times. Hot flushes and night sweats can negatively affect your quality of life, sleep, and overall well-being.

As a woman of God, remember you are salt, who is preserved, and adds flavour wherever you go; your lamp does not go out, but it burns on continually through the night of trouble, privation, or sorrow; warning away fear, doubt, and distrust. This is the visible influence the church is having in its area, Matthew 5:14-16.

A PRACTICAL TIP:

Dress in layers that you can remove easily if you begin to feel warm. Use lightweight sheets and blankets and wear loose, lightweight clothing to bed. Keep a spare towel nearby and be prepared to change into a fresh nighty. Use fans to cool your home, and keep a cool bottle of water by your bedside.

Note: A word of caution for those women who are considering using hormones to treat hot flushes and night sweats. Please pray and seek God's guidance first. Research has shown artificial hormones carry a risk of serious side effects and may not be safe for everyone. [Source: JAMA. 2002; 288(3): 321-333. doi:10.1001/jama.288.3.321]

A SHORT PRAYER:

Dear God, thank You for making me salt and light. I pray for supernatural healing. May others glorify You when they see my good deeds. In Jesus' name. Amen.

I decree and declare today: *"I am a woman of salt and light."*

DAY 14
ITCHY & CRAWLY SKIN
.V. DILIGENCE

♛

In her hand she holds the distaff

PROVERBS 31:19A

During menopause, a drop in estrogen levels can cause your body to produce less collagen and natural oils. This can cause your skin to become itchy.

Ever wondered why your hands may feel extremely dry and skin cracking immediately after washing them? Or do you notice a dry face when you look in the mirror? Itchy and crawling skin can cause discomfort and distraction during both work and relaxation.

As a woman of God, remember you are diligent in all you do; your hands hold the distaff, that is, the staff that the wool or flax is on before spinning. A distaff is designed to hold the unspun fibres. Therefore, you plan and prepare strategically, a structure for ministry teams of all ages, cultures, and different backgrounds to work well together, Acts 17:14-15.

A PRACTICAL TIP:

Avoid scratching. Carry a natural hemp hand cream in your handbag. Use one hundred percent certified aloe vera skin products. Take vitamin C supplements.

A SHORT PRAYER:

Dear God, thank You for making me conscientious. I pray against distractions, so I can plan the next steps in the work you have called me to steward. In Jesus' name. Amen.

I decree and declare today: *"I am a woman of diligence."*

Day 15
Electric Shock Under Skin
& in the Head .v. Useful

and grasps the spindle with her fingers.

Proverbs 31:19b

During menopause, many women experience a sudden sharp but short coursing of electricity through the body, similar to an electric shock.

Sometimes your scalp feels like something shooting underneath, or your fingers and elsewhere on your body can get a shock feeling. It can be a highly uncomfortable and painful feeling.

As a woman of God, remember you are plugged into The Messiah's Holy Spirit power; you lay your hands to the spindle. Spinning consists of the twisting together of drawn-out strands of fibres to form yarn. Therefore, you are twisting ministry teams together. A spindle is a straight spike, usually made from wood, onto which the fibre is being spun. This speaks about taking raw material and working with it until it becomes useful. So, you are teaching, training, equipping the church to do the works of ministry, Ephesians 4:11-12.

A PRACTICAL TIP:

Apart from providing you with the very much needed Vitamin D, natural sunlight will also soothe the nervous system helping you to alleviate electric shocks. Walking barefoot on natural flooring of sand or grass is also known to stabilise the nervous system.

A SHORT PRAYER:

Dear God, thank You for making me useful. I pray against attacks, so I can be effective in equipping the saints to be proactive in ministry. In Jesus' name. Amen.

I decree and declare today: "I am a woman of great use."

DAY 16

DEPRESSION .V. JOY

*She opens her arms to the poor
and extends her hands to the needy.*

PROVERBS 31:20

Depression is common during menopause and the post-menopause. Psychosocial factors also may increase risk of sadness during menopause.

Stressful life events such as a divorce, job loss, or the death of a parent are common occurrences for people in this stage of life. These events may trigger depression and you may find a lack of interest in once-enjoyable activities, or feelings of worthlessness, hopelessness, or helplessness. It can produce sudden despair and could bring back bad and sad memories, which then triggers further insecurities, anxiety, and depression.

As a woman of God, remember Christ has given you a garment of praise instead of a spirit of despair, Isaiah 61:3b. You open your hand to the poor, yes, you reach out your filled hands to the needy; whether in body, mind, or spirit, because you know to serve others, not only pleases God, it takes your mind off your circumstances, and proves to be rewarding, bringing joy and security, Proverbs 11:25.

A PRACTICAL TIP:

Take this pocket-sized devotional and read it daily; meditate on the scriptures. Feed your spirit by praying in tounges (if you have this spiritual gift – 1 Corinthians 14) for at least thirty minutes daily and take vitamin B supplements. Be careful what you watch, listen to, and be accountable to a trusted friend, who has your back, through prayer. Finally, go and help someone else, and watch how this will lift you out of self-pity.

A SHORT PRAYER:

Dear God, thank You for making me secure in Your love. I pray for Your presence to always be with me. I pray against the spirit of heaviness and ask You to replace it with a garment of delight, so that the joy of the LORD will be my strength, and I can reach out to the poor and needy with the Gospel and Your love. In Jesus' name. Amen.

I decree and declare today: *"I am a woman of joy."*

Day 17
Increase in Allergies
.v. Triumph

When it snows, she has no fear for her household;
for all of them are clothed in scarlet.

Proverbs 31:21

Falling oestrogen levels in menopause makes the body defend itself by producing more histamine, the powerful chemical that leads to allergy symptoms.

Some women develop asthma or eczema symptoms later in life. Ever wondered why you are suddenly sensitive to different environments like cold temperatures and air conditioning, or foods like nuts and gluten, or injections into your body like insect bites and pharmaceutical interventions, or skin absorbents like latex gloves and beauty products? Menopausal changes within your body can trigger allergic reactions you never had in your earlier years. Allergies are a nuisance and can in some cases, become life-threatening. This could cause fear or worry and hinder some of your work and social activity, if not managed properly, which then, can trigger other mental health issues.

As a woman of God, remember you are whole and an overcomer in Christ; you fear not the snow period of lack or spiritual cold, especially during winter seasons for you and your family. You and all your household are doubly clothed in scarlet. Scarlet dye comes from crushing the cochineal beetle. Therefore, you are confident that 'your people' are saved. You and they are covered in the blood of Jesus; this is how you will triumph, Revelation 12:11.

A PRACTICAL TIP:

Nettle tea or capsules acts as a natural anti-inflammatory, that prevents the body from producing histamines. Vitamin E and local honey may also reduce inflammation. If your symptoms are severe, please see your GP or go to hospital. If you are asthmatic, take your prescribed inhaler as instructed by your doctor.

A SHORT PRAYER:

Dear God, thank You for helping me overcome every obstacle. Similar to how Lydia's household was saved and baptized in, Acts 16:11-15, I pray for the blood of Jesus Christ to cover me and my loved-ones for salvation, and my ministry for Kingdom advancement. In Jesus' name. Amen.

I decree and declare today: *"I am a woman of triumph."*

DAY 18
IRREGULAR & FLOODING PERIODS
.V. PURITY

She makes coverings for her bed;
she is clothed in fine linen and purple

PROVERBS 31:22

Between long periods, short cycles, spotting, and heavy bleeding, your menstruation during perimenopause may be generally irregular. They may not settle into any distinct pattern, especially as you get closer to menopause. This can be unsettling and frustrating.

You may wonder why your periods are flooding and you are having to wear darker clothes and cover your bed spread and mattress with an extra red or dark sheet to prevent staining. When bleeding is heavy, it may last longer, disrupting your everyday life. You may find it uncomfortable to exercise or carry on with your normal tasks. Heavy bleeding can also cause fatigue and increase your risk of other health concerns, such as anemia.

As a woman of God, remember you are pure; you make for yourself coverlets, cushions, and rugs (coverings) of tapestry. Your clothing is of linen, pure and fine, same as robes of righteousness, and of purple, such as that of which the clothing of the priests (royal and priestly robes) and the hallowed cloths of the temple were made. You are not a second-class citizen. Jesus said to the woman with the issue of heavy and continuous bleeding, *"Daughter, your faith has made you whole. Go in peace and be freed from your suffering,"* Mark 5:34. Do not feel ashamed, as you are God's princess, who mentors and ministers to other women in the area of purity, Titus 2:3-5.

A PRACTICAL TIP:

Eat vegetables rich in iron. Eat 80 per cent raw and organic food. If you are feeling constantly weak or fatigued, please see your GP. They may check to find out whether you have fibroids. If you are going to preach publicly or minister, be sure to dress in your purple underwear and outer-clothing. Take plenty of extra sanitary products in your hand bag and change just before your speaking engagement slot.

A SHORT PRAYER:

Dear God, thank You for what Your Son Jesus Christ did on the Cross. He exchanged my filthy rags and gave me righteousness instead. I pray I will not see myself as unclean because You made me clean, and created me to stand for You, as my covering, so I can teach others to do likewise. In Jesus' name. Amen.

I decree and declare today: *"I am a woman of purity."*

Day 19
Tingling in the Extremities .v. Respect

Her husband is respected at the city gate,
where he takes his seat among the elders of the land.

Proverbs 31:23

Extremities are parts of your body which are far away from your heart. Oestrogen, one of the primary hormones in flux during menopause, has a complex effect on the central nervous system. When this hormone is thrown off balance during menopause, it can affect the nervous system, producing symptoms like tingling extremities.

You may be curious why areas of your body, including your bottom keep tingling. The irritating sensation can cause you to want to hit, rub or scratch those areas. This can be embarrassing and distracting in life.

As a woman of God, remember Christ respects you and your earthy husband is not ashamed of you, as you unapologetically, proclaim the Gospel around the globe. Neither is the heart of Your heavenly groom, Jesus, far from you, as He is known in the cities, towns, villages, communities, when He sits among the elders of the land, Luke 9:26.

A PRACTICAL TIP:

Eating a balanced diet, getting regular exercise and sufficient sleep can help.

A SHORT PRAYER:

Dear God, thank You for showing me respect and teaching me how to submit to others out of reverence for Christ, especially my husband. In Jesus' name. Amen.

I decree and declare today: *"I am a woman of respect."*

Day 20
Headaches .v. Integrity

She makes linen garments and sells them,
and supplies the merchants with sashes.

Proverbs 31:24

The hormone changes that happen as women approach the menopause mean that all types of headaches, including migraines, become more common.

You may notice you have been experiencing sharp stabbing pains in your head, or a dull ache in the background. Headaches can disturb your overall sense of wellbeing and slow you and your life down.

As a woman of God, remember you wear the helmet of salvation; you make fine linen garments and lead others to buy them; you speak the reality in love; offering salvation to others, through evangelism. You put on the full armour of God every day, and teach others integrity. You deliver to the merchants, belts of truth, or sashes that free one up for service, Eph 6:14.

A PRACTICAL TIP:

Avoid or cut down on dietary triggers of headaches which include alcohol, aged cheeses, caffeine, chocolate, and dairy products.

A SHORT PRAYER:

Dear God, thank You for being honest with me through Your word. Thank You for helping me point people to Christ, as my life, as well as my doctrine, is a witness. I pray I will always be truthful to others, in love, and behave in a conscientious way regardless of who is watching. In Jesus' name. Amen.

I decree and declare today: *"I am a woman of integrity."*

Day 21
Incontinence, Upon Sneezing & Laughing .v. Dignity

She is clothed with strength and dignity;
she can laugh at the days to come.

Proverbs 31:25

Urinary incontinence (UI) is also known as "loss of bladder control" or "involuntary urinary leakage," common in menopausal aged women.

You might only leak a few drops of urine when you laugh, sneeze, cough, or exercise. Or you might experience a sudden urge to urinate and be unable to keep it in before reaching the toilet. This can be soul destroying and rob your self-esteem.

As a woman of God, remember you may become even more undignified than this, as you dance unto the LORD, 2 Samuel 6:21-22. Strength and dignity are your clothing and your position is strong and secure. You gracefully rejoice over the future; the latter day or time to come, knowing that you and your family (the Ekklesia) are in readiness for it, Revelation 19:7.

A PRACTICAL TIP:

Wear the appropriate panty liners and do pelvic floor exercises, to strengthen your pelvic muscles.

A SHORT PRAYER:

Dear God, thank You for clothing me with dignity. I pray for You to continue to empower me to preach the word; be prepared in season and out of season. And in doing so, I am ready for the coming of our LORD! In Jesus' name. Amen.

I decree and declare today: *"I am a woman of dignity."*

Day 22
Dizzy, Light-headed & Loss of Balance .v. Wisdom

She speaks with wisdom,
and faithful instruction is on her tongue.

Proverbs 31:26

Hormones play an important role in balancing your blood sugar levels. Hormone changes during menopause affect how your body responds to insulin. Changes to blood sugar levels can make you dizzy. Also, changes in estrogen and progesterone, are known to affect your inner ears, which are critical to your sense of balance.

You may sometimes feel unsteady on your feet or feel like the room is moving or spinning when it is not. You might feel as if you are in motion when you are not moving. This can be scary, especially if you are in a place where you need to be focused or alert, due to the potential dangers around you, like crossing the road, walking up some steps, or driving. Also, if you are losing your coordination, often, others may think you are not fit to make sound decisions, or you yourself may believe this.

As a woman of God, remember you ask for wisdom when you lack it; you open your mouth in skillful and godly understanding, and on your tongue is the law of kindness; giving counsel and instruction wherever you go, Judges 4:4-8.

A PRACTICAL TIP:

Try drinking water and staying hydrated. Take vitamin D-3 supplements and add apples, ginger, carrots, and beetroot to your daily diet.

A SHORT PRAYER:

Dear God, thank You for giving me wisdom. I make wisdom my sister and understanding my closest friend, Proverbs 7:4. I pray for more understanding, discernment, and direction in all the decisions I make for Your glory. In Jesus' name. Amen.

I decree and declare today: *"I am a woman of wisdom."*

DAY 23
IRREGULAR HEART BEAT
.V. OVERSEER

*She watches over the affairs of her household
and does not eat the bread of idleness.*

PROVERBS 31:27

During the menopause it is common to notice heart palpitations or irregular heartbeats where it feels like a pounding or fluttering in the chest.

You may sometimes feel your heart skipping beats and the pounding feeling can radiate from your chest all the way up into your neck and throat. This can make you feel nervous about what is going to happen next and anxious about your overall health. You may feel the answer is to automatically stop working and exercising, which as a result, might be detrimental to the smooth running of your business and household.

As a woman of God, remember Christ's heart beats for you; you look well to how things go in your household, and the bread of idleness (gossip, discontent, and self-pity) you will not eat. As a protective mother-hen, you guard against little-foxes trying to intrude and destroy your God-fearing household. You always look for the next step or thing to do for the glory of God, 1 Timothy 3.

A PRACTICAL TIP:

Manage your blood pressure, blood sugar, and cholesterol levels. Maintain a healthy weight. Work hard for the LORD, but keep in step with the Holy Spirit, who would not cause you to burn-out.

A SHORT PRAYER:

Dear God, thank You for giving me the ability to work hard for Your Kingdom's extension; overseeing, but still allowing my husband to be the head of my household. I pray You will also help me set Godly boundaries; to have boldness to say 'no' to work You have not given me. Help me to know when to rest but not be idle. In Jesus' name. Amen.

I decree and declare today: *"I am a woman who oversees."*

Day 24
Breast Tenderness
.v. Blessings

Her children arise and call her blessed;

Proverbs 31:28a

Breast pains are a common part of the menopause transition, although they are experienced in different ways. For some women, it is an experience of tenderness, burning or soreness.

For those women who have given birth to a child, you may sometimes feel the similar pain to when you were breast-feeding your baby. This can be uncomfortable and, in some cases, unbearable.

As a woman of God, remember you are weaned on His love; your children rise up and call you blessed. They are healthy, due to the rich properties which came from your breast milk. They call you happy, fortunate, and to be envied because you, to them, are the best mum in the world, Psalm 131:2.

A PRACTICAL TIP:

Use evening primrose oil and wear a supportive sports bra when exercising.

A SHORT PRAYER:

Dear God, thank You for my physical and spiritual children. I pray You will bless them as they are a blessing to me. In Jesus' name. Amen.

I decree and declare today: *"I am a woman who is blessed."*

DAY 25
INCREASE IN FACIAL HAIR
.V. PRAISES

her husband also, and he praises her:

PROVERBS 31:28B

During menopause, a woman's body stops circulating estrogen but continues to circulate the same amounts of testosterone. The imbalance of hormones causes the appearance of some male secondary sex characteristics, like coarse facial hair.

Most women detest any sign of hair on their face, including fine hair. So, to have thick hair appearing can make a woman lose confidence in her appearance and femineity. Feeling insecure can sometimes be a distraction in work and life.

As a woman of God, remember your husband (King Jesus) boasts about you and praises you. He cannot stop speaking well of you; in fact, He sings over you and His banner over you is love, Zephaniah 3:17.

A PRACTICAL TIP:

Use a battery-operated, hand-held epilator, which removes hairs from the roots safely.

A SHORT PRAYER:

Dear God, thank You for praising me. I pray I will learn to receive Your praise and the praise of my earthly husband. In Jesus' name. Amen.

I decree and declare today: *"I am a woman worthy of praise."*

Day 26
Tinnitus: Ringing in Ears .v. Discernment

♔

"Many women do noble things
PROVERBS 31:29A

Oestrogen underpins signaling from the ears to the brain and falling levels during menopause, may be responsible for a mix-up in sounds being communicated between the two, leading to unwanted, inner ear noise.

Tinnitus is an internal, occasional, or continuous ringing, in one or both ears, with different pitches. But the noise is unique for each person, so for yours might be an engine sound, or high-pitched whine. Whatever you hear, is it any wonder that it can make life feel unbearable? Especially when it happens as you try to get some sleep. This can be very frustrating when trying to communicate clearly and be part of a conversation.

As a woman of God, remember, '…nor is His (God's) ear too dull…' to hear your cries for your wellbeing and your loved-ones, Isaiah 59:1. Many daughters have done virtuously, nobly, and well, with the strength of character that is steadfast in goodness, like Deborah, and you learn from her, Judges 5:2–31

A PRACTICAL TIP:

Exercise helps flush out excess stress hormones, boosts feel-good endorphins, and may distract you from fretting about your tinnitus.

A SHORT PRAYER:

Dear God, thank You for helping me be sensitive to sound and for giving me discernment for spiritual awareness. I pray I will not compare myself to others but rather learn from other women of God who have gone ahead of me, as I take note of their noble character and not allow my age, or condition to prevent me from being a strategist for You. In Jesus' name. Amen.

I decree and declare today: *"I am a woman of discernment."*

DAY 27
BARRENNESS .V.
HUMBLE SURRENDER

but you surpass them all."

PROVERBS 31:29B

As mentioned, you have not officially reached menopause until you have gone a whole year without a period. Studies suggest, once you are postmenopausal, your hormone levels have changed enough that your ovaries may not release any more eggs. Therefore, most women can no longer get pregnant naturally – BUT GOD!

Other than In Vitro Fertilisation (IVF), if it has been a year since your last period, you may consider yourself beyond your childbearing years. This can be a let-down for Christian woman who marry later in years, and feel broody, then regret not having the experience of giving birth to a baby. This could be a distraction from life, if you decide to look at alternate methods to having a child and unsure about the moral consequences.

As a woman of God, remember you have the humility of Christ; by faith even like Sarah, who was past childbearing age, was enabled to bear children because she considered Him (God) faithful who had made the promise, you too, can put your trust in God for that, which is not, as though it were. Sarah became the mother of all nations; so, will you, spiritually, as you wait on the LORD for His direction, and minister to people, including children of all races and cultures. You do not feel the need to compare yourself with any other lady, because you excel them all, Hebrews 11:11.

A PRACTICAL TIP:

Spend more time in humble prayers to God. A woman can only receive what is given to her from heaven, John 3:27. God can see the end from the beginning and He knows what is best for you, your husband, family, life, and ministry. If you still want children, practice surrender and long suffering. Read the stories of Sarah, Hannah, and Elizabeth in the Bible, who all conceived naturally and gave birth to heathy and God-fearing sons in their older age.

Finally, remember the scripture verse: Then Naomi (name means: gentle) took the child and laid him on her bosom, and became a nurse to him, 1 Ruth 4:16 (NKJV). Naomi was an old woman, and had not recently given birth to a child of her own. However, she breastfed her grandson. The scriptures indicate that Naomi did something equally important to the physical part – she spiritually breastfed her grandson. I urge you therefore, to embrace your role as a spiritual mother, to feed younger women in the faith, with the word of God, until the Church hands back the batten to Israel, before the time of Jacob's Trouble. See Jeremiah 30:6-8, Daniel 12:1, Matthew 24:15–31, and 1 Thessalonians 4:16, Romans 11:25-26.

A SHORT PRAYER:

Dear God, thank You for helping me to be gentle, and humbly surrender to Your perfect will for my life. But God; nothing is impossible for You! I pray, only if it is Your will, I will have a healthy, God-fearing child safely in my older age, for Your glory. Help me also to nurture my spiritual children. In Jesus' name. Amen.

I decree and declare today: *"I am a woman who humbly surrenders."*

Day 28

Thinning or Loss of Hair
.v. Inner Beauty

Charm is deceptive, and beauty is fleeting;

Proverbs 31:30a

Androgens production in menopausal women, shrink hair follicles, resulting in hair loss on the head.

Most women experience overall hair thinning rather than noticeable bald spots. The thinning can occur on the front, sides, or top of the head. Hair may also fall out in large clumps during brushing and showering. The Bible says, whenever a woman grows her hair, it is a glory to her, 1 Corinthians 11:15. There is nowhere in the Bible, where it states that thick hair is the best. However, hair loss, for many women can knock confidence. It can also be another distraction from life, if you worry and spend too much time looking for wigs and extensions.

As a woman of God, remember you are beautiful inside and out; charm and grace are deceptive, and beauty is vain, because it is not lasting. This is like a church that looks great outwardly, but what is actually going on the inside? Do not be like the church of Sardis? Revelation 3:1-6.

A PRACTICAL TIP:

Drink a cup of green tea during the first half of the day, can help. Also try and keep your hair natural. Your beauty should not come from outward adornment, such as elaborate hairstyles and the wearing of gold jewelry or fine clothes. Rather, it should be that of your inner self, the unfading beauty of a gentle and quiet spirit, which is of great worth in God's sight, 1 Peter 3:3-4.

A SHORT PRAYER:

Dear God, thank You for my inner beauty. I pray I will not be deceived by the vain trimmings of the worldly standards. Help me to be content and transformed by the renewing of my mind, for Your glory, Romans 12:2. In Jesus' name. Amen.

I decree and declare today: *"I am a woman of inner beauty."*

Day 29
Grey & Silver Hair
.v. Admiration

but a woman who fears the Lord is to be praised.

Proverbs 31:30b

As you age, your hair can also become gray as it loses melanin. This of course, is not an issue confined to only females, however, menopausal women, would have experienced some change of hair colour by this stage of their life.

The Bible says, gray hair is a crown of splendor; it is attained in the way of righteousness, Proverbs 16:31. As we age, the gray hairs represent the wisdom we have gathered over the years and should be admired. However, most women desire to keep the hair colour of their youth; while others, would do anything to change their natural colour through dying. If you allow negative thoughts about gray hair to take root, it could rob you of the joy of knowing who you are in Christ, no matter how you look. Sadly, I have noticed how a few women in ministry, who have made a lot of money, use their riches for plastic surgery, silicone breasts, and other excessive artificial coverings, which gives the impression, they are wearing a mask.

As a woman of God, remember you are admired by Christ; you are like the church of Smyrna and Philadelphia, who receives only praise and her crown guaranteed, from our LORD, Revelation 3:10.

A PRACTICAL TIP:

As previously mentioned, drinking green tea can help maintain melanin in your body. The fear of the LORD is the beginning of wisdom. To illustrate the point that God loves you just the way you are, read my book, 'You Fit Perfectly', and meditate on the scriptures reinforcing who you are in Christ.

A SHORT PRAYER:

Dear Abba Father, thank You for Your admiration and for filling me with Your Shekinah Glory. I pray I esteem others, by telling them about what is to come upon this world, in the hope they will repent before the rapture. I pray also, I will stand firm in my faith, so no-one will take my crown, Revelation 3:11. In Jesus' name. Amen.

I decree and declare today: *"I am a woman to be admired."*

Day 30

Osteoporosis
.v. Double Honour

Honor her for all that her hands have done,

PROVERBS 31:31A

Osteoporosis can be a symptom of menopause at a later stage. This is where your bones begin to weaken. If you fall when your bones are in this state, they may not be strong enough to sustain the fall, and they may fracture. If osteoporosis is severe, fractures can occur even without a fall or other trauma.

No Kingdom-minded woman, whether single, married, divorced, or widowed, wants to be out of action for long, so it is understandable for women who suffer from bone frailty, to be concerned about injuries in later life. The Bible says, Do you not know? Have you not heard? The Lord is the everlasting God, the Creator of the ends of the earth. He will not grow tired or weary, and his understanding no one can fathom. He gives strength to the weary and increases the power of the weak. Even youths grow tired and weary, and young men stumble and fall; but those who hope in the Lord will renew their strength. They will soar on wings like eagles; they will run and not grow weary, they will walk and not be faint, Isaiah 40:28-31.

As a woman of God, remember you are honoured. You will see the fruit of your hands and receive double honour, as your onlookers (those disciples who have gone before you), cheer you on, as you fix your eyes on Jesus, the perfector of your faith, Hebrews 12:1-2.

A PRACTICAL TIP:

Both calcium and cod liver oil, can help build strong bones and keep them strong as you age. Keeping fit also helps prevent bone loss.

A SHORT PRAYER:

Dear God, thank You for double honour. I pray Your word over me: "Instead of your shame you shall have double honor. And instead of confusion they shall rejoice in their portion. Therefore in their land they shall possess double; Everlasting joy shall be theirs", Isaiah 61:7 (NKJV). In Jesus' name. Amen.

I decree and declare today: *"I am a woman of double honour."*

EXACERBATION OF EXISTING
CONDITIONS .V. PERSEVERANCE

and let her works bring her praise at the city gate.

PROVERBS 31:31B

Menopause can aggravate existing health issues such as diabetes, asthma, chronic obstructive pulmonary disease (COPD), weight gain, fibromyalgia, insomnia, attention-deficit hyperactivity disorder (ADHD), autism, obsessive compulsive disorder (OCD), bipolar, and depression.

If you are at the stage where you receive more concerns from the medical practitioners about your blood test results, or you feel like you are suffering from multiple health conditions all at once, you are not alone. It may seem unfair, get you down, and you may question God about why, after doing so much work for your family, community, church and in some cases, the nations, He is allowing you to struggle in the area of health. God the Father will never leave you; Jesus is your best Physician, and His Holy Spirit is your wonderful Counsellor. The LORD will not give you more than you can bear, 1 Corinthians 10:13.

As a woman of God, remember Christ has not finished with you yet. Others are still looking to you for advice, Godly counsel, guidance, and intercession, which you can do anywhere you are located and whichever position you find yourself in. Remember you live in a fallen world; you are only passing through this earth, 1 Chronicles 29:15, and you will eventually be given a glorious everlasting body, 1 Corinthians 15:35-58! Halleluiah! Jesus will let your own works praise you in the gates of the city, where you live and where you may pass away to be with Him, to hear those precious words, "Well done [daughter], good and faithful servant! You have been faithful with a few things; I will put you in charge of many things. Come and share your Master's happiness! Matthew 25:23.

A PRACTICAL TIP:

At this stage, you may require some professional intervention. However, hold onto the Apostle Paul's words: "I have fought the good fight, I have finished the race, I have kept the faith. Now there is in store for me the crown of righteousness, which the Lord, the righteous Judge, will award to me on that day—and not only to me, but also to all who have longed for his appearing," 2 Timothy 4:7-8.

A SHORT PRAYER:

Dear God Almighty, thank You for perseverance. I pray I will run in such a way as to get the prize. Everyone who competes in the games goes into strict training. They do it to get a crown that will not last, but we do it to get a crown that will last forever. Therefore I do not run like someone running aimlessly; I do not fight like a boxer beating the air. No, I strike a blow to my body and make it my slave so that after I have preached to others, I will not be disqualified for the prize, 1 Corinthians 9:24-27. So, help me God. In Jesus' name. Amen.

I decree and declare today: *"I am a woman of perseverance."*

LIST OF REFERENCES

onlinemenopausecentre.com

healthline.com

evernow.com

mymenopausecentre.com

nhs.uk/conditions

positivepause.co.uk

jamanetwork.com/journals/jama/fullarticle/195120

narikaa.com

aafa.org

menopausecentre.com.au

jwa.org/encyclopedia

Meet the Author

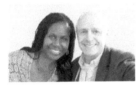

Tope Pearson, is Patron to The Precious Foundation, Co-Founder of Equipping the Saints Ministries, a Speaker and Author of many books including Debt Revelation – Do Not Look Back; You Fit Perfectly; Why are you Running?; The Cry of a Londoner; The Wedding Dress; Heal to Health; The Lonely Soldier; Finding your way out of the Menopause Maze; and You Fit Perfectly for Kids. She has also written song lyrics and poetry.

All of Tope's books are available at www.youfitperfectly.co.uk or via leading online bookstores including Amazon and Barnes & Noble.

Tope is married to Tim Pearson and they have six children and seven grandchildren in total. They both speak on subject matters for equipping the believers.

For more information, please go to their website: www.etsministries.org.uk

Milton Keynes UK
Ingram Content Group UK Ltd.
UKHW022129150424
441110UK00002B/1